# A HEALTHIER AND LONGER LIFE

AMAZING WEIGHT LOSS GUIDE MADE EASY WITH
SUSTAINABLE MINI LIFESTYLE CHANGES FOR
BEGINNERS. A MUST HAVE FOR EVERY WOMEN!

## H. A. SKYS

# CONTENTS

# INTRODUCTION

*It frustrates me when I see advertisements and statements like: "lose weight in 20 days" or "get in shape in 7 minutes every day" or "drink this chemically compounded product to lose weight," diet plans that promise us we will lose 30 pounds in 6 weeks, and the list goes on. Who knows the long-term health issues they may cause you!*

*As we all know, these quick fixes don't work in the long-term. If they did, we would ALL have the ideal body weight/shape we have dreamed of all our lives.*

*You're reading this book because you have tried different diets, different weight loss programs, and unfortunately they never quite worked for you. I know it can be one of the most devastating things to experience. You might have been left feeling that there is no hope for you, and even worse, hating your body.*

*Most women understand that weight loss requires a mixture of healthy eating and working out regularly. But what happens if you're doing all the right things but rather than losing weight you are actually gaining weight, or you are not seeing the results of all of your hard work. Do not fear nor worry. This book will explain and explore some possible reasons why you are gaining or have gained that weight.*

*You will learn techniques and tips which will give you natural and sustainable results that will last a lifetime. Some ideas on losing weight you may be already aware of, but implementing them with other techniques and tips will result in astounding weight loss.*

*You would be amazed how simple lifestyle changes can aid your weight loss. This could make the world of difference - no stress and no pressure, as no one is perfect, after all. If you slip up one day, don't be hard on yourself, just go back onto it. Eventually you just keep on doing the simple mini changes, and before you know it, it becomes part of your everyday lifestyle.*

*As every day in every way you are doing better - yes you can, yes you will and yes you have!*

*This book has been compiled after a great deal of research, finding out about new scientific facts and reports studying weight gain and obesity. This information can help you finally discover why you are the weight you are or why you have recently gained weight. With the help of this book, you will be advised on everyday useful lifestyle changes, tips, and techniques to shed the weight and keep it off for life.*

*Are you ready to unlock the hidden secrets that you may be aware of or may not be aware of or even once knew but have completely forgotten? Better yet, combining different elements together could result in greater and faster weight loss. This book will go through your genetics, your environment, your method of eating, physiological reasons and so many more different elements will be looked into.*

*You've got it in you to achieve any goal and overcome any obstacle life throws at you just as long as you have the correct information and guidance. Anything is possible! It's time to claim that body you've always wanted, that has always been there, just waiting for you to unleash your true potential, your true you.*

*If you keep on taking the same actions for two weeks, it becomes second nature, it becomes your habit, it becomes a way of life.*

# HOW TO USE THIS BOOK

*First, complete the following task called "Before you start,_think, write, and do the following." Once you have completed that task, it's vital to go through this book chapter by chapter. Answer the questions as and when they are applicable to you, which are marked as "To think about/to do" and can be found at the end of each chapter. Make physical notes of your answers on a new, unused notepad or journal. Don't take any immediate action until the end of the book, as it is important to obtain all the information first before deciding on what mini changes you should look into first.*

*Before you start, think, write, and do the following:*

**1.** *Write and underline the following title at the top of your notebook or journal "My Future Body".*

**2.** *Why do you really want that body?*

*Write at least three reasons.*

**3.** *Imagine yourself with your idea of your ideal body. What would you look like? And what changes would you make to your life because of it?*

*Write at least five answers.*

**4.** *Get a full-length picture of what you think the perfect body you want looks like. This could be of anyone and any picture size, just as long as it fits on your notepad or journal (you could always fold the picture so that it fits). Then stick it on the next page of your paper notepad or journal. The picture you choose should be a realistic and achievable goal for you to aim for.*

*Mark / name this picture "My Future Body".*

# 1

# WHY BEING OVERWEIGHT OR OBESE
# A REAL PROBLEM

## WORLD HEALTH PANDEMIC

*E*xperts have reported that they have seen a staggering rise in levels of obesity over the last 46 years. A large proportion of the world's population is either overweight or obese or even morbidly obese. There are various factors that contribute to someone becoming overweight and obese, like slow metabolism, genetics, culture, bad nutrition, overeating, and even lack of the correct amount of sleep. Food combinations and the actual time of the day in which food is consumed can also have a major impact on your overall weight and quality of life.

*In a study by "World Health Organization, in June 2021" announced that in 2016, there was more than 1.9 billion adults from the age of 20 were overweight. 650 million adults were classed as obese. A staggering 39% of the adult population was classed as overweight. More than 380 million children and teenagers between the ages of 5-19 was obese or overweight. It is known that obesity kills more people than being underweight does. Surprisingly, there are more overweight and obese women than men in the world.*

*The more excess weight we carry day in and day out, the more our lung capacity is lowered, meaning it is harder to get oxygen into our major organs and around our body. This has an immediate impact on our heart functionality. We are putting unnecessary and constant pressure on our entire body. Around 2.8 million people die yearly from being overweight or obese, and that amount is rising every year.*

*The percentage of obesity in the population varies in different countries due to the availability of consumable foods and lifestyles. A country's overall monetary status has no link to its obesity rate. However, wealthier countries have a greater ability to advise people on what they are consuming.*

*In research conducted in 2021, countries were listed by the highest to the lowest obesity rates. Here are some results.*

## THE 3 COUNTRIES WITH THE HIGHEST OBESITY RATE

*1st place:* *Nauru Island, located in the southwestern Pacific Ocean, ranked as the world's 1st placed country with the highest obesity rate at 61%.*

*2nd place:* *Cook Island, located in the south Pacific Ocean, north-east of New Zealand, ranked as the country with the 2nd highest obesity rate in the world at 55.9%.*

*3rd place:* *Palau, located in the southwest corner of Micronesia, ranked as the world's 3rd-highest obesity rate at 55.3%.*

## THE TOP 3 COUNTRIES WITH THE LOWEST OBESITY RATES

*1st place:* *Vietnam, located in Southeast Asia, ranked as the world's 1st placed country with the lowest obesity rate at 2.1%.*

*2nd place:* *Bangladesh, located in Southern Asia on the Ganges River, ranked as the world's 2nd-lowest obesity rate at 3.6%.*

**3rd place:** *Timor Leste, located at the eastern end of Lesser Sunda Island, ranked as the world's 3rd placed country with the lowest obesity rate at 3.8%.*

*The number one spot of countries with low obesity rates is Vietnam. But they have a larger number of people that are extremely underweight. They have launched support to promote better lifestyle choices for people in their city locations where obesity is high and are also addressing the issues of undernourishment for their citizens based more in village type locations.*

*The number one spot for the highest-ranked country with obesity is Nauru. Their typical diet is mainly high sugar soft drinks, carbohydrate-heavy foods, and non-fresh food. This has also resulted in a high rate of type 2 diabetes and other health issues related to obesity in that country.*

*A study was conducted in "2020 by Bloomberg Global Health Index" researching which countries are the healthiest in the world. They considered factors like great healthcare, low pollution, safe drinking water, quality of life, and lifespan.*

## BELOW ARE THE TOP 5 HEALTHIEST COUNTRIES IN THE WORLD

**1st place:** *Spain. Out of a score of 100, Spain scored 92.75. The expected lifespan is 83 years, and this will increase in years to come. They are a country* *of walkers, with almost half of the people that live there walking regularly. Their diet consists mainly of fresh fish, fresh fruits, fresh vegetables, and a very low amount of processed food.*

**2nd place:** *Italy*
**3rd place:** *Iceland*
**4th place:** *Japan*
**5th place:** *Switzerland*

*Being or becoming overweight or obese can increase your risk of developing serious health conditions and complications. The general definition of someone being overweight or obese is when one has an excessive amount of fat that could cause health issues like the following, but only to name a few:*

- *Some types of cancer*
- *High risk of having a stroke*
- *Type 2 diabetes*
- *Heart disease*
- *Gallbladder disease*
- *High blood pressure*
- *High LDL and Low HDL cholesterol*
- *Osteoarthritis*
- *Sleep and breathing problems*
- *The ability to conceive a baby and/or carry to full term becomes more difficult*

- *Depression, anxiety and other mental health disorders*
- *Mobility issues*
- *Low self-worth*

*In general, adults from the age of 20 years old and above are considered obese if their body mass index is above 30.*

## BMI WEIGHT CATEGORIES AND CALCULATION

*1.85 to 24.9 BMI means you are at a healthy weight*
*25 to 29.9 BMI means you are overweight*
*30 to 39.9 BMI means you are obese*
*40 and above BMI means you are morbidly obese*

*The most commonly used technique to check your BMI is to make the following calculations:*

1. *Step on to a scale and take a note of your body weight in kilograms (kg).*
2. *If you don't know your height already, get a measuring tape and measure your height in metres (m).*

*Then do the following: Your Weight (kg) divided by your height (m); once you have the answer, then divide by your height again.*

## For example:

*A woman that is 85 kg in weight with a height of 1.70 m.*

*The calculation would be: 85 divided by 1.7 (do not include the last zero from your height number) then press the equals button (=) to give you the answer (50). 50 divided by 1.7 (height again) gives you the answer 29.41 BMI, which shows that this woman would be categorised as overweight.*

*Remember, a female's BMI is to be used as overall general information, as it does not tell a person's fat-to-muscle ratio. It also does not take account of your ethnic background.*

*Being overweight or obese is very common and very serious. But with the correct information and simple lifestyle changes you can reduce and maintain your weight, which can indeed last a lifetime.*

## TO THINK ABOUT/TO DO

*It's important to know your personal body mass index BMI as a guide. We advise that you calculate your BMI by following the above calculations and make a note of it on your notepad/ journal and mark the day's date next to your BMI score.*

*Don't be alarmed by whatever number your BMI calculation produces.*

*This is only chapter 1, you have so much more information to consume and analysing to do. So please move onto the next chapter to increase your knowledge.*

# 2

# THE ROLE OF GENETICS IN WEIGHT GAIN

## YOUR GENES AND YOUR WEIGHT

*G*enetics *is a study showing how different qualities, called traits, are passed down from our parents. Each parent gives you one chromosome each which creates 46 chromosomes in total. It helps to explain what makes you, you. Why do some diseases run in some families and not in other families? Why do we look like our siblings and even our grandparents?*

*When we investigate our genetic makeup and its qualities, we would be looking at the information called genes. As humans, we have trillions of cells. 99% of the cells in your body have a nucleus, where all your genes are located. We all have different sets of genetics - even twins. No two people in the world have the exact same set of genes. Genes are like a blueprint of your body, from how your body is structured to how it carries out day-to-day functions.*

*With regards to your weight, there are a number of genes that could cause a tendency to be overweight or obese. Genes play a huge role that could cause one to overeat and consume a high number of calories to feel satisfied. While someone with a different genetic makeup would eat a much smaller number of calories and feel satisfied. It has been found that genes account for about 70% of the variation in a person's body weight.*

*As individuals, we all have a set-point weight range. This is the range your body deems as "normal" for your genes and body type. In other words, normal when you're eating a healthy balanced diet without restriction and working out without overdoing it. If you try to dramatically reduce your weight in a short amount of time, by eating much too little, signals will be sent to your brain, causing it to react by pushing your weight to the size it considers to be the correct body weight for you. As a result, many people experience weight gain after undergoing the latest diet craze or long-term and excessive exercise programs.*

## TEST: ARE YOUR GENES AFFECTING YOUR WEIGHT?

*Your genes might be affecting your weight, especially if one or more of the following are true for you*

> *Q1) Do you eat healthy foods and work out regularly but cannot seem to lose weight?*
>
> *Q2) Are other members of your family overweight or obese? Are your parents overweight or obese?*
>
> *Q3) Would you say that you have been experiencing weight issues for most of your life?*

**If you answered yes to one or more of the above questions, then you are more likely to have a genetic tendency to be overweight or obese. You will be more likely to experience weight issues yourself. In fact, the probability is as high as 75%.**

*On the other hand, it is highly unlikely your weight issues are caused by your genes if one or more of the following traits are true for you:*

> *Q1) Have you experienced hitting a plateau in your*

*workout routine, then you changed it and started to see the weight coming off again?*

***Q2)*** *Would you consider yourself to be slightly over-weight and can see more weight loss when you commit to a new diet or workout routine?*

***Q3)*** *Do you tend to go for healthier food choices in general?*

**If your answer was yes to more than one of the above questions, then you would be less likely to have a genetic tendency to be overweight or obese.**

## COMMON GENE

*There is a type of gene called thrifty genes. This is a very common type of gene which more than 80% of the world's popu-lation has. The thrifty genes enable individuals to collect and process food to deposit fat during food abundance to provide for periods of food shortage. Thrifty genes also slow the rate of metabolism, making it harder to lose weight, but not impossible.*

*There are other genes that are known to cause people to be over-weight or obese, as they influence the way we feel after we eat, our appetite, our body composition, glucose adsorption, and so on.*

## OTHER COMMON GENES

**Ankyrin B**: *Makes fat cells that absorb glucose at a very fast rate.*

**MC4R**: *The Melanocortin 4 Receptor affects our metabolism by regulating the levels of energy we use from what we have eaten and notifies us when we are feeling hungry.*

**IRX3**: *The Iroquois homeobox gene 3 is the gene that may make it more challenging to lose weight.*

**The FTO**: *People with this gene have a 30 percent higher chance of being overweight. This is a protein gene that is linked to fat mass.*

*Do you have any of the above 5 weight-gaining genes? Knowing the answer to this question would make it easier to know what works best for your body to achieve your weight loss goals.*

*With that said, women with a low to moderate genetic tendency to being overweight or obese can still lose weight. Eating the correct foods that are specific to your metabolism type and sticking to a regular workout plan would aid your weight loss rather than gain. It is going to take a lot of time, effort, and willpower to achieve your desired weight. Go slowly, meaning aim to drop 10 to 15% of your body weight every 6 months, until you get to your ideal body weight.*

*Your genes do play a major part in your physical development. They can determine your height, your athletic ability, your intelligence level, and much more. Because your genetic makeup plays a part in your weight and body type, you can still make changes to your weight. The first important step to take is to educate yourself. You can even do a DNA test at home to find out your genetic makeup and to see what type of weight-gaining genes you might have.*

*But don't be mistaken - you are not a slave to your genetics. It is how you use your DNA testing results that truly matter to your overall weight loss success.*

## TO THINK ABOUT/TO DO

*Please answer the above questions as truthfully as possible and make a note of the results in your journal so that you can refer back to them at the end of this book.*

*When it's time to start making mini lifestyle changes, just remember that Rome wasn't built in a day. Go slowly so your brain doesn't fight back to result in what it truly believes is your correct weight.*

This is only chapter 2, you have so much more information to consume and analysing to do. The next chapter will help you gain even more understanding about what makes you gain weight.

# 3

# UNINTENTIONAL LIFESTYLE CHANGES THAT CAN MAKE YOU GAIN WEIGHT

*Unplanned weight gain is an extremely common event that can happen to all of us. There are lots of causes of unintentional weight gain. If you noticed that your favourite jeans or that dress that normally complements your figure all of the sudden does not. Rather than fitting in all the right places, it's hard to even get the button on. Or your shapewear seems to be literally suffocating you. You may feel like you are doing all the right things, like eating healthy and working out, so what in the world is going on! There are other reasons you need to consider that could explain why you are piling on extra pounds.*

*Have you personally and recently experienced any of the following changes in your life within the last year?*

## NEW RELATIONSHIP

*New love? It can equal weight gain. You may think "who cares I'm in love" - but you will. It's natural to go out to restaurants as a new couple, meeting each other's families and friends, which may result in eating and drinking more than you would normally. Or the complete opposite - you stay in binge-watching the latest Netflix or Amazon prime video. With all this newness, the last thing you are thinking about is healthy eating or working out. Why would you? You've got your partner now, life is great, and you just want and need to spend as much time as possible with each other.*

*Then that love weight starts to creep on. You find yourself holding that stomach in and hope he or she has not noticed the bulge. Months later you are asking them "do you still love me?" and "do you still find me sexy?"*

*New relationships are amazing, but don't forget who you are and were before you fell in love. Find fun and active activities that you and your partner might enjoy together.*

**Remember, it's so easy to gain weight, but twice as hard to lose.**

## STARTING A NEW JOB

*Surprisingly starting a new job could lead to weight gain, for example:*

- *If you are moving into a new career or industry that could add additional stress.*
- *If your journey into your new work location is less active and takes longer, and you find yourself sitting down for longer periods. Or even worse, your new role involves you only working from home.*
- *If you find the workload overwhelming, and it's stressful and hard to manage.*

## BEING PREGNANT

*As we all know, not all pregnancies are the same, nor all pregnant women. For example, it's very different being pregnant in your twenties compared to being pregnant in your forties, trust me! No matter what age you are, what is guaranteed is weight gain (or, as I called it, keeping the baby warm). Depending on the weight you were before you conceived, as a rule, you should try to keep your weight gain to an additional 25 to 45 pounds (this also depends on the weight of your delightful baby bump). If you're carrying more than one baby, this must also be taken into consideration. The key is not to put on too much weight, as of course, it would make it harder to lose the weight after childbirth. After giving birth, particularly if you're breastfeeding, is not the best time to start a diet plan (as we know diets only lasts for a period and not for a lifetime). You would also have to make sure that you are eating enough calories, which would be about the same number of calories you were consuming before you gave birth.*

*Eating enough calories is not just important for you, but it's also important for producing breast milk.*

*Remember the old wise saying "nap and sleep when the baby naps and sleeps"? Well, this is so true and one of the best bits of advice I has ever been given when I was a first-time mother. As we know, sleeping has so many health benefits and is one of the top requirements for women, especially after giving birth.*

## STARTING COLLEGE OR UNIVERSITY

*It has been proven that around 75% of university and college students gain weight, especially during the first year. This is due to various reasons, like change in sleeping pattern, very late nights, social eating and drinking and lack of money (which equals cheaper and unhealthy food choices). Furthermore, new experiences could be overwhelming and stressful. When you combine at least two of the above elements, it's no wonder the pounds are just piling on.*

*The best method to keep from adding on more weight is to keep an eye on it by regularly weighing yourself using scales twice a week and writing down your weight. Also, it's advisable to reduce your alcohol intake, and not to drink it too late as it affects your quantity and quality of sleep.*

*Just like any new change in life, it just takes some time to get used to it.*

*The key is to find ways to be more active, no matter what situation you find yourself in.*

## TIPS

1. *Do you find yourself sitting down for a long period on your way to work, school or university? Or when you are at work, school or university, you're unable to leave your desk? If so, try doing heel taps, ankle stretches and rotations.*
2. *See if you can make your way to work, school or university on a bike, all the way or partway.*
3. *Get up from your desk and walk faster to the toilets and back to your desk.*
4. *If you are working from home, or find you are at home more often than normal, exercise on your way to the toilets and kitchen or do some desk workouts.*
5. *Every hour or so that you are sitting down for a long period of time, do a 1-minute exercise (each time focus on a different part of your body).*
6. *Go for a walk (power or speed walking) at your lunch break.*
7. *For a cheaper and healthier lunch, make food from home to bring into the office to have for lunch.*

*Find creative ways that suit and fit your personal circumstances.*

## TO THINK ABOUT/TO DO

*Over the last year, have you experienced any of the above unintentional lifestyle changes that made you gain weight? If so, take a note of it. Are there any other unlisted unintentional lifestyle change that made you gain weight? If so, take a note of it.*

*Remember what was said in chapter 2? When it's time to start making mini lifestyle changes, don't forget that Rome wasn't built in a day. Go slowly so your brain doesn't fight back to result in what it believes is the correct weight for you.*

*This is only chapter 3, you have so much more information to consume and analysing to do. The next chapter will give you even more knowledge.*

# 4

# HOW AGING MAY AFFECT YOUR WEIGHT

## MY LIPID TURNOVER

*N*ew scientific research has confirmed why people gain weight the older they become. As we age our bodies do not respond in the same way to weight loss as they used to. On average, some of us can gain weight, but not all of us. We tend to gain 1 to 2 pounds every year, and there is a reason for that.*

*That reason is called lipid turnover. Good news - now some of us can say "It's not me it's my lipid turnover!" Lipid turnover is the balance between triglyceride storage and removal. Lipid turnover in our fat tissue reduces the older we become, and it doesn't even matter if we are not actually eating more than we used to. As a result, so many of us can find it hard to maintain our weight the older we become thanks to lipid turnover.*

*It has been discovered that lipid turnover processes fat tissues completely independently, meaning no other factors contribute to this. This is great news, as scientists are getting a better understanding of lipid turnover and its various mechanisms. Due to the worldwide obesity epidemic, it's even more important to understand how lipid turnover affects the storage and removal of lipids.*

*It has been reported, but not proven, that one way we could speed up our lipid turnover in our fat tissues is to increase the number of workouts we do.*

*Just because we are getting older should we stop caring about our health and our body confidence? Have you heard the following statements? "It's normal," "I mean, you are getting older." No, don't listen to any of that noise. In fact, not every single older person will gain weight. Some do and some don't. Here's your chance to say "Nope not me, not today! I was cute in my 20s and in my 30s, and I will be cute at any age!"*

**Here are some tips you can add into your life to get back into shape and maintain it for years and years to come.**

## PROTEIN

*Helps build and strengthen muscle mass, so eat lean protein with every meal. The following foods are high in protein: lean red meat, fish and seafood, skinless chicken breast and turkey, greek yoghurt, cottage cheese, eggs, tofu, vegan meat alternative products such as quorn, protein powder, nuts, seeds, legumes, and beans. Protein-rich foods can also keep hunger at bay because it's more satisfying and keeps you fuller for longer.*

## YOUR "6 A DAY"

*Yes, I said it - your 6-a-day. Why not opt for an increased amount of the recommended intake? Fruits and vegetables should be fresh or frozen, never in a tin that has been sitting on the supermarket shelf for who knows how long. Tinned fruits and vegetables are packed with preservatives, sugar or syrup, or sweeteners, and they are a no-no. Fresh or frozen fruits and vegetables are packed with vitamins, potassium, minerals, and folate. They will also give you the all-important fibre, which supports gut health and prevents digestion issues. When it comes to which ones to purchase, think of all the colours of the rainbow. Avoid those you have allergic reactions to and intolerances.*

## WALKING

*The underestimated value of walking! Here are some of the health benefits of walking. It improves our lung and heart functionalities, which reduces the chance of developing heart disease and experiencing a stroke. It improves our balancing ability and helps to build bone strength. It can also help to manage conditions like high blood pressure, high cholesterol, joint and muscular pain, or stiffness.*

*So don't pick up your car keys! Get your trainers or comfortable footwear and just walk. Walk to the shops, walk around the house. Walk in the park, slow walk, and then pick up the speed and power walk. Don't use the elevator; rather choose to walk up the stairs or downstairs. Walk with wrist or ankle weights. If you're not accustomed to walking, you soon will be. Just take it easy at first and extend the length of time you walk and your speed each time. It's recommended that you do meaningful walking at least four times a week.*

***Remember what I mentioned about the world's healthiest country? That's right, Spain is the number 1 country for walkers.***

## STRENGTH/WEIGHT TRAINING

*Strength training has been well documented to be extremely beneficial to us. No matter your age, you could even be in your eighties (with guidance and the correct method), as it builds and retains your muscle mass. Muscle cells burn calories at a quicker speed than fat cells, and it increases your metabolic rate.*

*Why weight training? This type of training is subjective to the individual. If you haven't weight-trained before, you should always start light. At first, start with a 0.5 to 1kg set of dumbbells. You could even try workout bands, which are used more in resistance training but also target the muscle. There are tons of options to choose from, but stick to those appropriate for your level of fitness.*

**It's recommended that you contact your doctor or health expert before starting any new workouts, to remain on the safe side.**

## TO THINK ABOUT/TO DO

*What new habits would you consider? Note them down in your book or journal.*

*When it's time to start making mini lifestyle changes, don't forget that Rome wasn't built in a day. Go slowly so your brain doesn't fight back to result in what it believes is the correct weight for you.*

*This is only chapter 4. You have so much more info to consume and analysing to do. So please move on to the next chapter.*

# 5

# MENSTRUAL CYCLE

## THE MONTHLY CHANGES

*O*n my period, aunt flow, my visitor, that time of the month, on my monthlies, code red, girl flu. The correct terminology is menstrual cycle, period, or menstruation. A new international report found that there are over 6,000 different slang terms and euphemisms for a women's period.

*On average, women gain about 3 to 6 pounds during their period, and some women experience the weight gain a week before their period is due to start. It can take up to one week for the weight gain to go away again, but on average 3 to 4 days during your period. This type of weight gain is due to hormonal fluctuations. It may be caused by overeating, missed workouts due to stomach cramps, water retention, and sweet cravings. I will go into more detail below.*

*You can also expect PMS, Premenstrual Syndrome, which comes with a wide range of different behavioural, physical, and emotional symptoms. Some women experience PMS from one to two weeks before their period even starts. It's caused by hormonal changes in your body and is extremely common, as more than 93% of women who have periods also have PMS.*

*Why must we have to go through so much as women? I hear you wondering.*

### *Here is a list of changes and explanation as to why:*

- *When you're experiencing stomach cramps due to your period the last thing you want to do is to put any pressure around that delicate area. So understandably, you might skip one or two or three workout days.*
- *You might experience a heightened sense of hunger and cravings, which could result in extra weight gain.*
- *When your due to come on your period, do you feel more tired with less energy than normal? This is due to the increase in your progesterone and estrogen levels. This can start to happen seven days before your period is due to start.*
- *GI - Gastrointestinal: Some women can experience issues such as abdominal pain/cramps, diarrhoea, or*

constipation. *Seven days before your period starts your progesterone level gets higher and your intestinal muscle weakens. The result of that would slow digestion rates and then lead to constipation.*

- *You may temporarily suffer from abdominal and pelvic pain due to prostaglandins. Prostaglandins make your uterus contract and shed your uterine lining, which results in starting your period. This natural process can be especially painful for some women. Others don't experience any pain whatsoever.*

**A lot of women have some of these symptoms before, during and after their period.**

**Advice No 1**: *Have to hand as much healthy food you truly enjoy around and during that period, so when cravings start you are prepared. Make sure it's a healthier option that does not have added sugar, syrup or sweetener.*

**Advice No 2:** *It has been reported that walking during your period is the best way to reduce menstrual cramps without putting too much pressure on your body. So, ladies, drop the medication and try walking. I know walking is the last thing you want to do, but try it, as you might be pleasantly surprised.*

*Advice No 3:* *For additional ease to stomach cramping and pain, you can find numerous resources online that focus on specialised yoga or stretching routines for women during their menstrual period.*

*Removing and adding certain types of food to your diet can improve menstrual-related symptoms.*

## FOOD YOU SHOULD AVOID WHILST MENSTRUATING

*Food intolerance: Most of us already know what type of food we have a non-life-threatening allergic reaction to or have an intolerance to, but love nevertheless. We try our hardest not to consume them on a regular basis, but if we are being honest with ourselves, we do treat ourselves to them now and then. But it's advisable not to treat yourself to those types of foods during your period, as it could make your symptoms much worse.*

*Meat: For all the fellow red meat lovers - although we all know red meat has health benefits, such as being high in iron, do stay away from red meat during your menstrual cycle, as it's high in prostaglandins which causes stomach cramps.*

*Lower your sugar intake: A bit of sugar never hurts, but just a small amount of sugar. If you tend to feel emotionally low during your period, taking a high amount of sugar could make your mood worse during your menstrual cycle. A high intake of sugar equals weight gain.*

**Say no to alcohol & coffee**: *Don't panic, it's not forever, only during your period! Why? Alcohol and coffee can trigger and/or worsen period symptoms, such as digestive issues linked to nausea and diarrhoea. You can also become dehydrated from drinking alcohol and coffee, which can make you even more bloated and can cause migraines. Coffee contains caffeine, and some of us drink more than we should in a day. It's recommended to reduce the amount of coffee consumed in a day dramatically or - even better - not to have any coffee during your period, if possible. Coffee has been linked to water retention during your menstrual cycle. Alcoholic beverages are full of calories and sugar which can lead to weight gain.*

**Sodium/salt**: *Bloating and weight gain are also triggered by foods with high amounts of salt/sodium added to them. As we all know, processed foods have the highest amount of salt, so it's recommended to reduce your salt intake and stay away from processed food whilst you are on your period.*

*But there is some good news!*

## FOOD YOU SHOULD DEFINITELY CONSUME WHILST MENSTRUATING

**Fresh Fruits**: *Fruits that are naturally sweet, which will help your desperate urge for sweet food, and they level out your glucose* *level. For good hydration, eat fruits that are high in water during your period. For example, cucumber is 96% water and has the highest water content of any food. Cantaloupe, which is in the melon family, is 90% water. Other melons are also good during your period. Strawberries are made up of 91% water. A Peach is made up of 89% water.*

*Always drink plenty of water! Of course, we all know the importance of drinking water in general, but you should drink even more water during your period, as it reverses dehydration, water retention, headaches/migraine, bloating and could also reduce the number of days your period last for.*

***Green leafy vegetables****: They are high in iron, magnesium, and various types of vitamins. They can help with the feeling of dizziness, tiredness, and muscular pain. The best green leaves to have during your monthly cycle are kale, spinach, watercress, collard greens, and beet greens.*

***Superpowers of ginger****: You can get the benefits of ginger in several ways. You can let the raw ginger simmer in a pot of boiling water and then drink it hot, or drink ginger tea or even just eat it fresh and raw. Ginger is one of the go-to natural remedies for periods and even during the first stage of pregnancy. Ginger can help relax aching muscles and it can also help with nausea. When you're feeling tired, consume ginger to get a natural boost of energy.*

***Omega-3s and fish***: *Fish is packed with beneficial Omega-3 fatty acids and protein, and it can relieve period pain dramatically. It also helps to balance your emotions during your period. It could also even help with facial breakouts during menstruation. As fish contains protein, it will also help prevent you from feeling the need to snack, which will reduce weight gain during your period.*

*The following period-related symptoms may or may not contribute to weight gain due to your period. These symptoms may occur while you are on your period, before or even after your period:*

- *Low sex drive*
- *Sweet food cravings*
- *Increased appetite*
- *Disturbed sleeping pattern*
- *Breakouts of spots or pimples*
- *Sore and or heavy breasts*
- *Mood swings making you easy to anger*
- *Depression and/or anxiety*

*You may not have experienced any of the above symptoms, or you may have experienced a combination of them. You might also experience them when you get older.*

***Magnesium supplements***: *These could be a great help, as they can improve the following: help to reduce PMS symptoms,* *regulate the nervous system, increase energy levels, improve muscle movement, help with protein formation, help to fight depression, may reduce inflammation and headaches.*

***Fish oil supplements****: These can help with weight loss and can reduce fatty liver tissues. They might also reduce inflammation, help with skin health, and help to balance emotional symptoms. They might also help with age-related mental decline and with bone health.*

*Fish oil supplements are not recommended if you have fish allergies or intolerance.*

*Always speak with your dietician, health advisor or doctor before taking any supplements.*

*Your periods and all the physical and emotional symptoms that come with them are normal! We as women are a wonderful and fascinating species, highly resilient and extremely strong mentally and physically.*

*But we are not all made exactly the same.*

***If you suffer from very painful period pains or long periods where you are bleeding constantly for more than 7 days, please speak to your healthcare professional or doctor, as there may be underlying health issues.***

## TO THINK ABOUT/TO DO

*What menstrual symptoms do you personally experience regularly? Have a good think about it and make a note of your symptoms in your book or journal.*

*How do your eating habits change before, during and after your period? Please make a note of any changes.*

*What changes would you consider making before, during and after your period to improve your symptoms? Please make a note of them.*

*This is only chapter 5, you have so much more info to consume and analysing to do. So please move onto the next chapter.*

6

# THE BENEFITS OF THE HUMBLE
# WATER

*H2O is the chemical symbol for what we know as water. Water is a compound of oxygen and hydrogen, which we regularly consume in a liquid form. It is the most vital compound in its natural form, with no odour or taste. Water is necessary for all chemical reactions that occur in living cells. Water is located everywhere on earth, the moon and even thought to exist on other planets. It is present in the oceans, rivers, rain, clouds and, of course, our bodies. Water comes from natural sources that are either groundwater or surface water. All living organisms are mainly made of water, around 60% for humans, between 80-90% for plants and 80% for fish.*

*As we all know, drinking water every day is vital for overall good health, regardless of the temperature outside. Water can improve your energy levels, and it's also been reported that it aids better brain function. But surprisingly a lot of people are actually dehy-*

drated. *This is particularly true for adults, as the older you get, the less sense of thirstiness you feel, in comparison to younger people.*

*The role that water plays is the following: balances your sodium levels, supports your digestive system and transports oxygen and nutrients to your cells. Water also controls your body temperature from overheating, regulates heartbeat, supports functionality to your organs, aids supple joints and maintains a healthy bladder.*

## BENEFITS OF DRINKING WATER FOR WEIGHT LOSS

*Apart from all the health benefits that drinking water brings, it can also support weight loss. Drinking hot water, in particular, helps to break down fat in the body and also mobilises it into molecules, resulting in it being easier for your digestive system to do it's job efficiently and burn fat.*

*It also works to reduce the amount of food you intake in one sitting, as it has been reported that drinking warm water can help you to reduce your appetite, resulting in eating less. It has also been shown that sometimes when you're actually thirsty, your body thinks it is hungry, causing you to overeat. In fact all it needed was a glass of water.*

**Tip**: *Drink a whole cup of warm to hot water (as hot as you can manage) 30 minutes before every meal.*

## WHAT COULD HAPPEN WHEN YOU DRINK TOO LITTLE OR TOO MUCH WATER?

*The cells in our body need water not just to function, but to function to their highest abilities for best health. Here are signs you can look out for that would indicate you are not drinking enough water and could possibly be dehydrated:*

*A feeling of weakness and confusion, dizziness and light-headedness, dry mouth, poor skin health, dark yellow and strong-smelling pee, peeing as little as four times a day.*

*As they say, everything in moderation is key! It can be alarming to know that something so good for you can also be extremely dangerous for you, if you don't implement moderation.*

*Drinking too much water is called overhydration, which can cause water intoxication. This happens when you consume too much water. This can lead to too much water in the brain cells, which results in swelling and pressure to the brain. If this continues for a long time, it could lead to developing high blood pressure or low blood pressure. Overhydration also lowers your salt levels (sodium) which imbalances the fluid in your cells. Untreated overhydration could cause serious health issues and conditions. It could lead to having liver disease, congestive heart failure and kidney problems, and even death, which is rare but not impossible.*

*It's worth noting, however, that overhydration from drinking water is extremely unlikely because the kidneys do such a good job of processing water. Overhydration is more likely to be caused by a problem in your body. Therefore, if you have recently experienced any of the following symptoms, you should consult with your doctor or health professional:*

*You may experience very frequent urination (more than 10 times a day), urine is clear in colour, weakening of muscles, headache, nausea, vomiting, unconsciousness or seizures.*

## WHAT'S THE CORRECT AMOUNT OF WATER TO DRINK?

*For many years the standard advice has been to drink 2 litres of water a day, which is equivalent to 8 glasses of water, as a general rule. However, this isn't 100 percent accurate. For example, compared to an adult, an eight-year-old child should not drink the same amount of water per day. It depends on your age, sex, body weight and your daily activities (workout). The amount of water taken in a day should vary from person to person and depend on each individual's circumstances. The current and the most accurate measurement to gauge the amount of water to drink would be by judging against half your body weight.*

***For example****: If your body weight is at 200 pounds, this means your goal would be at least 100 ounces each day, or 2.84 litres, which is roughly 12 cups of water per day. It's important to adjust the quantity by the circumstances and criteria mentioned above, to your personal lifestyle.*

## WHAT TO DO IF YOU DON'T LIKE THE TASTE OF WATER?

*You know the importance of drinking water, but for some reason you can't stand the taste of it.*

**Tip:** *Try infusing your water. Simply add natural fruits or vegetables to your water to your taste. For example, add slightly squeezed raspberries or blueberries to release the flavour. You can also try your water with a fresh slice of orange, lemon or lime. You can even try some vegetables in your water, such as celery or cucumber.*

**Weight loss advice:** *Adding fruits or vegetables to your water is also a great way to promote weight loss. Vegetables and fruits with high water content like grapefruit, broccoli and yellow melon are at least 90% water, watermelon and bell pepper are 92% water, spinach is 93% water, tomatoes 94% water, celery 95% water, and cucumber are 96% water.*

*As previously mentioned, drinking warm to hot water 30 minutes before meals is beneficial for fat burning. When it comes to drinking water during the time that you are not eating a meal, ice-cold water has amazing benefits, including weight loss. Cold water helps to boost your metabolism rate because your body must work harder to warm it up as you drink it, resulting in burning more calories.*

*Consuming warm water regularly helps your body to break down fat deposits, relaxes your muscles and enhances blood flow. The increased blood circulation will rejuvenate skin cells and keep them nourished.*

*At night, your body naturally detoxes and repairs itself. This results in most people waking up feeling dehydrated and with a dry mouth. Drinking hot lemon water first thing on an empty stomach reduces a foggy brain, reduces bloating, promotes clear skin, improves circulation, and stimulates your bowel, allowing the body to remove waste easier and quicker.*

## INFUSED WATER RECIPES TO HELP WITH WEIGHT LOSS AND PROVIDE OTHER HEALTH BENEFITS

1. *Cold or hot drinking water with fennel seeds promotes weight loss and enhances the digestive system.*
2. *Hot drinking water with ginger reduces stomach bloating and cures colds and headaches.*
3. *Cold drinking water with cucumber and grapefruit helps with weight loss.*
4. *Hot water with peppermint tea reduces bloating.*

***This might come as a surprise, but not all water is made equally!***

## DIFFERENT TYPES OF WATER, THEIR BENEFITS, AND NEGATIVE ATTRIBUTES

**Alkaline water** has ORP oxidation-reduction potential. It also contains a higher pH level, which is higher than tap water.

> **Benefits**: As alkaline water is believed to have some additional benefits that are not yet actually proven. Some people believe that alkaline water is much healthier water to consume as they believe it can prevent cancer and keep you looking youthful.
>
> **Negatives**: When consuming large amounts of alkaline water, it has been reported that you can experience nausea and vomiting caused by metabolic alkalosis. Caution must be taken, as it could affect your stomach acidity, resulting in less ability to kill harmful bacteria. But when consumed in small doses, it is deemed safe to drink.

**Mineral water** is exactly what it says on the tin. Mineral water is packed with minerals, like calcium, sulfur and magnesium, which are great for your health.

> **Benefits**: The amazing benefit that mineral water provides is that it supplies our body with minerals that our bodies cannot produce naturally, as listed above. It also helps with our digestive system.

**Negatives**: *There have not been any reported negatives about mineral water, apart from the cost. But quality does not come cheap after all! Some mineral water has a high sodium content, so if you are on a low-sodium diet, you might need to check the label of the mineral water you choose to ensure you pick one with a low sodium count.*

**Distilled water** *is a processed water. The production of distilling water is as follows: water is boiled and when it reaches boiling temperature, the steam is literally gathered and converted back to water.*

**Benefits**: *Distilled water will be beneficial if you are in a location where the water supply is poor quality.*
**Negatives**: *It's not advisable to drink distilled water as a long-term option. It contains no minerals or vitamins, so could therefore obtain vitamins and minerals from your body or teeth.*

**Sparkling water,** *carbonated water, or soda water. Fizzy water is produced by mixing water with carbon dioxide gas with a high level of pressure.*

**Benefit and negatives**: *Sparkling water contains minerals that are good for your health. However, for weight loss purposes, avoid those with added flavouring,* *sugar or sweeteners. Some brands can also be relatively expensive.*

**The key to keeping yourself hydrated is to monitor and listen to your body and drink water every day.**

---

## TO THINK ABOUT/TO DO

*How much water are you currently consuming in a day? How do you plan to make your everyday water give you weight loss benefits?*

*Keep a track of your water intake in general. This can be easily done by downloading a free water tracker app on your phone.*

*When it's time to start making mini lifestyle changes, don't forget that Rome wasn't built in a day. Go slowly so your brain doesn't fight back to result in what it believes is the correct weight for you.*

*This is only chapter 6, so you have so much more info to consume and analysing to do. If you love smoothies, you won't want to miss the next chapter.*

# 7

# WHY SMOOTHIES ARE GOOD FOR WEIGHT LOSS

## THE IMPORTANCE OF SMOOTHIES

*Researchers have confirmed time and time again how freshly made smoothies are not only beneficial for your overall health, but can also slim down your waistline, decrease inflammation, support digestion, burn fat and drop your dress size. Not only are they very quick and simple to make, but they can also satisfy any taste buds. It has also been shown that your body absorbs the vitamins and minerals from your fruits, vegetables, seeds, yoghurts or milk, green powders, herbs and spices, green leaves, healthy fats, and nuts better when you liquefy them into a smoothie.*

*Smoothies can also be a meal replacement and makes it easy to drink your recommended five-a-day in one sitting. Of course, not all smoothies are equal! The ingredients for a smoothie for weight loss will be different than for a smoothie that is for promoting muscle gain. Combining the wrong ingredients can indeed pile on the weight, as some fruits are higher in sugar than others. With that said, we would not exclude all naturally high-sugar fruits completely, rather you will only use a small amount. It would be more effective to combine ingredients like "superfoods" that have protein, fibre, amazing flavour, minerals, vitamins, and antioxidants. They will aid weight loss and keep you fuller for longer. Smoothies can be consumed any time of the day, even first thing in the morning or in the evening. What you will need to consider is choosing ingredients suitable for the time of day. Certain ingredients could spike your energy levels, which would be the last thing you would want if you were due to go to bed shortly after consuming your smoothie.*

***For example**, if you have a smoothie in the evening, ensure you finish drinking it at least three hours before bedtime to give your body a chance to process it.*

*Smoothies are also time-saving, and you can prepare your smoothie the night before if you are short of time in the mornings.*

*Remember, it's still crucial to eat a well-balanced meal every day and not to consume only smoothies. Don't shy away from using frozen fruits and vegetables in your smoothie, as it could actually be more nutritious than fresh fruits and vegetables. Just look for frozen choices that have been picked and frozen immediately. We can also recommend that you portion out your smoothie ingredients the same day you purchase your fresh ingredients and freeze them to preserve the nutrition in them. The minute your fruit and vegetables are picked from the tree or ground, they will start losing their health benefits.*

## SMOOTHIE RECIPES FOR WEIGHT LOSS

*To follow are some smoothie mixtures that are really healthy for you, low in sugar and packed with nutritional benefits to help with your weight loss journey:*

### *KALE SMOOTHIE*

### *Ingredients:*

- *Kale 1/2 (half cup)*
- *Medium size banana 1/2 (half medium)*
- *Chia seeds 1/2 teaspoon*
- *Hemp seeds 1 teaspoon*
- *Organic spirulina powder 1 teaspoon*
- *Oat milk OR almond milk 1/2 (half a cup)*
- *Vanilla OR Plain Whey protein powder 1 scoop*
- *Water 1/2 (half a cup)*
- *Ice optional (2-3 cubes)*

***Preparation:*** *Add ingredients into a blender or nutribullet and blend to your desired thickness. Add chia and hemp seeds after blending.*

*Serving & Tips: One serving. Don't use any product that is labelled low-fat or low-sugar.*

## RED SMOOTHIE

*Ingredients:*

- *Cooked beets 1/2 (half a cup)*
- *Mixed frozen berries 1/2(half a cup)*
- *Ginger, small knob*
- *Plain yoghurt OR plain greek yoghurt 1/2 (half a cup)*
- *Oat milk OR almond milk 1/2 (half a cup)*
- *Ice optional (2-3 cubes)*

**Preparation**: *Add ingredients into a blender or nutribullet and blend to your desired thickness. Add water to blend (optional).*

**Serving & Tips**: *One serving. Don't use any product that is labelled low-fat or low-sugar. If you don't have frozen mixed berries use blueberries or strawberries.*

## GREEN SMOOTHIE

*Ingredients:*

- *Apple 1 (whole)*

- *Medium size Banana 1/2 (half medium)*
- *Pineapple 1/2 (half a cup)*
- *Plain whey protein powder 1 scoop*
- *Uncooked, washed kale 1/2 (half a cup)*
- *Uncooked, washed spinach 1/2 (half a cup)*
- *Oat milk OR almond milk 1/2 (half a cup)*
- *Ice optional (2-3 cubes)*

**Preparation***: Add ingredients into a blender or nutribullet and blend to your desired thickness. Add water to blend (optional).*

**Serving & Tips***: One serving. Don't use any product that is labelled low-fat or low-sugar. Don't remove the skin of the apple, just remove the seeds.*

## PROTEIN PUNCH SMOOTHIE

### Ingredients:

- *Cooked Black beans 1/4 (quarter cup)*
- *Avocado 1/2 (half medium)*
- *Banana 1/2 (half)*
- *Pumpkin seeds 1 teaspoon*
- *Oat milk OR almond milk 1/2 (half a cup)*
- *Cayenne pepper a pinch*
- *Plain whey protein powder 1 scoop*
- *Ice optional (4-5 cubes)*

**Preparation**: *Add ingredients into a blender or nutribullet and blend to your desired thickness. Add water to blend (optional).*

**Serving & Tips:** *One serving. Don't use any product that is labelled low-fat or low-sugar. The avocado should be soft and ripe, peeled and the seed removed. If you don't have any cayenne pepper, use any other hot sauce or dry hot pepper seasoning you have. Or you could also use turmeric instead, which has a wealth of health benefits, but without the hot kick.*

## FRESH SMOOTHIE

**Ingredients**:

- *Lime 1/2 (half)*
- *Grapefruit 1/2 (half)*
- *Celery 1 stick*
- *Ginger small knob*
- *Cucumber 1/4 (quarter)*
- *Water 1/2 (half a cup)*

**Preparation**: *Add ingredients into a blender or nutribullet and blend to your desired thickness.*

**Serving & Tips**: *One serving. Peel and remove seeds from lime and grapefruit. Don't remove the cucumber skin.*

## *TROPICAL SMOOTHIE*

### *Ingredients:*

- *Lemon 1/4 (quarter)*
- *Banana 1/2 (half)*
- *Mango 1/2 (half cup)*
- *Watercress 1 cup*
- *Oat milk OR Almond milk 1/2 (half a cup)*
- *Plain Whey protein powder 1 scoop*
- *Ice optional (2-3 cubes)*

**Preparation***: Add ingredients into a blender or nutribullet and blend to your desired thickness. Add water to blend (optional).*

**Serving & Tips***: One serving. Don't use any product that is labelled low-fat or low-sugar. Remove the skins and seeds from the fruit. As this smoothie is a bit high in natural sugar, only have ones a week.*

*It's recommended to have one-two servings of smoothie per day. We have sourced the healthiest smoothie ingredients, with low to medium natural sugar, creating weight loss boosting smoothie combinations for you.*

## TO THINK ABOUT/TO DO

*What smoothie do you currently consume each day?*

*Which of the smoothies suggested above will you consider adding to your life? Please make note of them in your note pad or journal.*

*When it's time to start making mini lifestyle changes, don't forget that Rome wasn't built in a day. Go slowly so your brain doesn't fight back to result in what it believes is the correct weight for you.*

*This is only chapter 7, you have so much more info to consume and analysing to do. So please move onto the next chapter, all about the benefits of teas.*

# 8

# TEA & HERBAL TEAS FOR WEIGHT LOSS

## THE GREATNESS THAT IS TEAS AND HERBAL TEA

*erbal teas, also known as tisanes, originated in China, then spread to Egypt, Japan and then to Europe and the rest of the world. Tea was believed to have medicinal properties. It has been recorded that the first cup of tea was drunk in 2737 BC. Herbal teas are made by decoction (removing the essence) or by infusion using edible plant material, herbs, leaves, tree bark, seeds, fruits, flowers, roots or spices.*

*Drinking herbal teas is another great way to promote weight loss. They can be extremely cost-effective and easily sourced. The majority of herbal teas contain catechins that can boost your metabolism and help your body break down fat quicker. Most herbal teas also contain caffeine which increases your energy levels, causing your body to burn more calories. They also have multiple health benefits.*

**Listed are the best three herbal teas to introduce into your life.**

## GREEN TEA

*The big wig of beneficial teas is your one and only green tea! Green tea does not only support weight loss, but it is also packed with antioxidants and substances that increase metabolism to help the pounds slip right off. Also, the caffeine found in green tea releases energy slowly without spiking and then dipping. It has been shown that if you drink 2 to 3 cups of green tea that is rich in catechins every day for a long period (an average of 1 to 3 months), it could actually change the formation of a person's fat gene components, reducing your stomach fat and overall weight loss. Green tea is also great for coffee lovers, as you can swap your coffee for green tea with no added sugar or milk. It can take around 7 days or so to get used to the taste, but it's extremely rewarding for your weight loss and overall health.*

## OOLONG TEA

*Second runner-up to green tea is the oolong tea. Oolong tea enables your body to produce heat from energy, resulting in burning off more calories (thermogenesis) and reducing the formation of new fat cells. Oolong tea is consumed once a day or twice a day.*

## PEPPERMINT TEA

*This tea is known to reduce bloating around the stomach area and can help cure sweet cravings. It has been scientifically proven that the aroma of peppermint triggers signals to the brain to reduce the sense of hunger. You can drink this peppermint tea after meals, but ideally at least two cups a day.*

## ADVICE

*Start with drinking green tea for the amazing health benefits and weight loss aid. It's recommended to only have 2 different herbal teas a day, 4 cups maximum in one day. For example: drink one cup of green tea in the morning instead of your coffee and another cup in the afternoon. In a day, and in addition to drinking two cups of green tea, you can also drink, two cups of either peppermint tea or oolong tea.*

## TO THINK ABOUT/TO DO

*What teas do you currently consume in a day?*

*Considering the teas mentioned above, which ones would you consider adding to your life? Please take note of them in your note pad or journal.*

*When it's time to start making mini lifestyle changes, don't forget that Rome wasn't built in a day. Go slowly so your brain doesn't fight back to result in what it believes is the correct weight for you.*

*This is only chapter 8, you have so much more info to consume and analysing to do. So please move onto the next chapter to see how stress and depression can affect your weight.*

# 9

# HOW STRESS AND DEPRESSION MAKE YOU GAIN WEIGHT

## WHAT IS STRESS?

*S*tress is the way in which humans process and react to unknown, unprepared and uncomfortable situations. Stress arises where someone may have been made to feel afraid, unsure, mentally or emotionally inadequate or have an overbearing feeling of being overwhelmed. Stress tends to have obvious and measurable triggers, such as running late for a meeting, going on a blind date, discovering you have a flat tire in the middle of nowhere. Small to moderate doses of stress can be beneficial to us, as it is a healthy and normal emotion, which we have all experienced. Stress, believe it or not, is key to human survival, but again only in moderation, as high levels and quantities of stress can be extremely dangerous to your health.

## WHAT IS DEPRESSION?

*Depression is also known as major depressive disorder. Surprisingly, depression can affect a lot of people without them even being aware that they are suffering from this illness. Depression is deemed to be a serious medical illness. There are currently 4 recognised different types of depression: psychological, existential, situational and biological. Depression affects the way you act, how you feel about situations and the way you process information. It can make even the happiest person feel extremely sad and lose interest in what was once a great passion for them.*

## HOW DOES STRESS AFFECT YOUR BODY?

*Stress affects your body through messages from the hypothalamus located in the brain which releases your stress hormones as a defence and coping mechanism. This results in a rise in your breathing speed and your heart rate, meaning your body goes into fight or flight mode. This is a normal reaction now and then, but it becomes abnormal if you feel this sensation numerous times in a day or almost every day. This could lead to severe health issues, like depression and anxiety.*

## HOW DOES DEPRESSION AFFECT OUR BODIES?

*Depression is a mental and physical illness. It can affect your entire body if it goes undetected and untreated for long periods. It can affect your nervous system, your memory and can cause delayed reaction in particularly in older adults, in comparison to younger adults. Depression can also dramatically affect your appetite and nutrition as well as your immune and cardiovascular systems. You may experience the urge for self-harm or suicidal thoughts or turn to substance abuse for some relief from your symptoms.*

## DOES STRESS AND DEPRESSION MAKE WOMEN PUT ON WEIGHT?

*Mismanagement or chronic stress can definitely promote weight gain. This is because your cortisol level becomes elevated, which in turn increases your appetite and naturally you experience weight gain. That couple of pounds, that stubborn fat that you cannot seem to get rid of, could be because of your cortisol holding on for dear life. I'm sure you're thinking that must be the worst of it, but sorry no! That dreaded cortisol also affects what part of your body you gain that weight increase. People with depression could experience loss or a gain in weight, depending on the type of depression, the length of time they have been experiencing depression, the type of medication they have been prescribed and how long they have been taking it for. Weight gain while being depressed would be due to the person's lack of motivation which results in an inactive lifestyle, consuming excessive food and in general, eating more comfort food rather than healthy foods. It has been reported that over 44% of adults who have been diagnosed with depression are also obese. Obesity and depression are linked.*

## SELF-TEST FOR STRESS

*Given below are some common symptoms of an individual that may be experiencing symptoms of high or chronic stress and depression.*

### *Symptoms of high or chronic levels of stress*

1. *Unconscious change to your eating habits*
2. *Concentration difficulties*
3. *Aches to the head and body*
4. *Insomnia*
5. *Frequent sickness*
6. *Feeling overwhelmed regularly*
7. *Problems with focusing*
8. *Experiencing memory loss*
9. *Irritability and being easy to anger*

## COMMON SYMPTOMS OF DEPRESSION

1. *Thoughts of committing suicide*
2. *Self-harm*
3. *Sleeping more or less than your normal sleeping pattern*
4. *Feeling negative about yourself*
5. *Lacking in hope and feeling sad*
6. *Always wanting to be alone*
7. *For no particular reason, losing interest in your regular activities and hobbies*
8. *Feeling aggravated, agitated or restless without understanding why*
9. *For no valid reason, experiencing rage and anger*
10. *Little energy and little motivation to do anything*
11. *Eating much more or much less than you normally do*

*Stress and depression can seem very similar and in some cases do have similarities, but they are also very different. Some people can actually be experiencing depression and have been experiencing it for some time and not even be aware of it.*

*With regard to normal levels of stress related to normal life events and triggers, it's easier to understand and acknowledge. Stress is not classified as a mental health illness as it naturally resolves itself in a short space of time. However, stress can definitely be a gateway to developing depression if the stressful situation continues for some time without any resolution. Since 2017, research by the National Institute of Mental Health found that at least 17.2 million adult Americans had experienced at least one episode of depression.*

## THERE ARE 4 DIFFERENT TYPES OF HAPPINESS CHEMICALS

**Dopamine, oxytocin, serotonin and endorphins.**

*Those happiness chemicals and hormones affect your environment, relationship, diet, sleep and workout plan. You have the ability to influence your mood, your choices, and actions you take each and every day. If you are feeling stressed out, you can see it affecting your life.*

## TIPS AND TECHNIQUES

*1. Move more, do more physical activities like walking, jogging, and exercising. As this is a great way to release endorphins, aka the happy hormone, it also helps your sleep quality and length and reduces your stress levels, which is a win-win.*

*2. Be at peace with yourself by meditating. There are lots of free meditation apps you can download onto your phone to help. You can search the internet for meditation, like YouTube videos. You can even search for more specific meditation, such as "meditation for reducing stress." Meditating from 10-30 minutes per day can bring great health benefits.*

**3.** *Find your inner calm by practising deep and relaxing breathing techniques. When practised correctly it will relax your muscles and supply your organs with more oxygen. Practise when you feel like you need to release stress and tension during the day and at night.*

**4.** *Use the power of laughter to release happy hormones and also reduce stress. Watch a funny film or programme. Find more shows featuring your favourite comedian and watch them all. Let yourself laugh and laugh until you cannot laugh anymore, until your cheekbones start to hurt, until you find it hard to breathe. Laughter is medicine for the soul. Which should be practiced as often as possible.*

**5.** *Socialise, go out with friends, visit family. Sit in the park and people watch.*

**6.** *Put your favourite music on and just dance. Dance like your life depends on it! Get lost in the music and feel that bass.*

**7.** *Affirmations can be very powerful, so write positive affirmations and stick them in places where you always see them. Practice saying them to yourself or out loud. Look in the mirror when you say them to really believe them.*

**8.** *Talk to a stranger. There are so many different support lines where you can talk to a professional free of charge about how you're feeling and why you think you are feeling the way you feel. Investigate what services you can get access to. Research and find a counsellor that you feel comfortable with.*

*The key to this is finding what feels good for you and you only.*

*Managing your stress today could stop depression from coming tomorrow.*

**Health is wealth!**

## TO THINK ABOUT/TO DO

*The self-test for stress or depression above is extremely important. Write down any symptoms that you are experiencing. If you find that you have more than two or three symptoms mentioned in the depression test and have been experiencing this for more than two weeks, consult your doctor or health professional to request a full assessment and seek treatment if necessary. It's always better to be safe than sorry. The above self-test should be used as a guideline and if you have any concerns at all, you should consult a doctor or other mental health professional.*

*If you know of anyone in your life that you believe may be suffering from clinical stress or depression, have an honest conversation with them. Let them read this book. Help them seek professional advice and let them know you are there for them and you care.*

*If you have two or more common stress symptoms, from the self-test. Refer to the tips and technique section to help lower your stress levels.*

*What stress-reducing techniques do you practice already? What new tips and techniques are you going to imple-*

*ment in your life? Please take note of this in your book or journal.*

*This is only chapter 9, you have so much more info to consume and analysing to do. So please move onto the next chapter.*

# 10

# HOW SMOKING AND SECOND-HAND SMOKE CAN AFFECT YOUR BODY WEIGHT

*P**eople started smoking tobacco as early as 3000 BC in South America. In the 17th-century tobacco smoking was introduced to Eurasia by European colonists. Towards the end of the 1920s scientists from Germany discovered the link between lung cancer and smoking tobacco, which then led to campaigns highlighting the risk of smoking.*

*Cigarettes are made from over 7,000 chemicals. When smoking cigarettes endorphins and dopamine are released due to the chemical reactions in a person's nerve endings. Consuming tobacco and getting that nicotine high is not just by smoking it, people can also sniff and chew it. You can get nicotine patches and electronic nicotine delivery systems.*

Some people start smoking as young children, mainly due to witnessing their older peers or via social media or being exposed to it in their homes.

Smoking negatively affects almost every part of your body and almost every organ. Smoking can cause and increase the chances of developing the following diseases and health issues: lung disease, chronic obstructive pulmonary disease, cancer, heart disease and stroke, blood clots, diabetes, some types of eye disease, rheumatoid arthritis, immune system, and crohn's disease. Some heavy and long-term smokers could need limbs amputated because of poor blood circulation.

Research has shown that a smoker's life span is reduced by 10 years in comparison to a non-smoker. The World Health Organization (WHO) announced that cigarette smoking is responsible for more than 5 million deaths every year.

Smoking has a detrimental impact not only on the smoker, but also on our planet, plants and animals, as it releases toxins into the air we breathe. The residue from cigarettes and cigarette butts sinks into the ground and waterways, resulting in water and soil pollution.

Recent studies concluded that a smoker may have better control of their overall weight. However, heavy smokers have an increase in abdominal and visceral fat, meaning having a popping, protruding stomach.

## SECOND-HAND SMOKE

*Alarmingly, it has been reported that inhaling second-hand smoke by non-smoking adults causes over 41,000 deaths a year, and over 400 deaths a year in children that are also exposed to second-hand smoke every year. Similar to the diseases found in smokers, second-hand smoke causes lung cancer, coronary heart disease and strokes in adults. Children and infants that are exposed to second-hand smoke can also experience the following: extreme cases of asthma, lung development issues, respiratory symptoms, ear disease and have a high risk of sudden infant death syndrome. Not surprisingly, pregnant women that are exposed to second-hand smoke could also find congenital issues in their babies and health complications during pregnancy, affecting both themselves and their unborn child.*

*Passive or second-hand smoke is more serious than we might realise. Even if a smoker smokes in a different room from non-smokers, or even if doors and windows are open, it would not immediately get rid of the toxic chemicals from cigarette smoke. The fumes from cigarettes can last in an enclosed environment, on furniture, on clothing and your hair for up to 8 hours.*

*Around the world, smoking is one of the leading causes of preventable death. Some people find quitting smoking more chal-lenging than others. The amazing health benefits of quitting smoking can start as quickly as a matter of hours after stopping. Many women are deterred from quitting smoking due to weight gain. However, weight gain as a result of quitting smoking doesn't always happen. Cigarettes contain nicotine which speeds up your metabolism resulting in your body using energy quicker, which burns calories at a faster rate. When you quit smoking your metabolism does the reverse. It will decrease and you could find yourself eating everything in sight, resulting in possible weight gain, especially if you replace the urge to smoke with food. As you might expect, weight gain can vary from person to person. It has been reported that within the first three months of quitting smoking, the risk of weight gain is extremely high. After the first three months, the speed of weight gain will normally reduce.*

*To succeed in quitting smoking for life you will need to have a plan in place to beat the nicotine craving and triggers.*

## AVOID PUTTING ON WEIGHT AFTER QUITTING

By doing the following:

***Advice 1) Reduce your portion size***: *Rather than having three big meals a day, try having four or five small meals a day. The difference is your portion size should be half of your normal size meal. Give yourself 25 to 30 minutes after you finish your meal and if you still feel hungry, then have a healthy snack as mentioned below. Eat small portions every three and a half hours and snack in between if you need to.*

***Advice 2) For keeping food cravings at bay****: You can help this by snacking on healthy foods in between meals. Snacks should not contain any added sugar, syrup or sweetener. Choose healthy options such as your favourite fruits, nuts or sliced vegetables like carrots, cucumber, celery and bell peppers.*

***Advice 3) Feed your metabolism****: Choose workouts that do not overly exhaust you. If you over-exercise it could make you hungrier, so stick to moderate-intensity workouts for a total of 2 hours every week over a whole week. So, do a workout every other day, or pick up your speed when walking. Aim to walk three hours per week, which is fast walking 30 minutes every day.*

***Advice 4) Get support****: There are plenty of different methods on the market to help you stop smoking, like patches, chewing gum, nicotine lozenges, counselling and even hypnosis.*

***Advice 5) Medication as the last result****: Seek advice from a professional such as your doctor, if you feel you need more support. There are medications available to help you stop smoking. But this should be the last result, as such medications will have side effects.*

## TO THINK ABOUT/TO DO

*No one should smoke for their whole lives as that is not a great quality of life to have. Why not stop today rather than tomorrow? Take the first steps. Remember smoking is a habit, a highly addictive one. Let us create better habits for our lives, before it is too late, as in the long run smoking is truly not worth it.*

*Remember that you can do anything that you put your mind to.*

*Do you personally smoke or have someone close to you that smokes? If you are a smoker, think about why you smoke. Given all the information about smoking and second-hand smoke I have just given you, is it really worth it as a whole? Have a think about what smoking does to our environment, our bodies, our families and the other people around us. Take a note of your answers in your note pad or journal.*

*This is only chapter 10, you have so much more info to consume and analysing to do. So please move onto the next and final chapter.*

# 11

## WE ARE TRULY WHAT WE EAT

*long with oxygen and water, food is one of the most important essential elements for all living humans to consume. Food provides the nutrients you need to build new cells for growth and to repair your body. It provides the energy required to keep you alive and active throughout the day. Healthy, well-balanced food keeps you healthy and prevents infections and diseases. It also provides good brain functionality and healthy organs. The type of food we eat every day has an effect on the nutrients we receive to keep us alive and healthy.*

## HEALTHY FOODS

Consist of the following components:

*Healthy fats, carbohydrates, protein, vitamins and minerals. But not all foods are the same, some have more and some have less beneficial factors. Furthermore, food can affect our mood, our sleep and so many other elements in all areas of our lives. If you consume too much or not enough food, you can become overweight or underweight.*

*So, when we say you are what you eat, we really mean you are what you eat! Your body is made up of all the things you consume. In addition to the types of food we eat, we are also affected by the time of day we eat. The type of food you consume and when you eat them both play a part in your overall body weight.*

*Researchers have concluded that it is not just what you eat that needs to be considered when it comes to weight loss, it's also when you eat. So, the time of day in which you eat can make a huge difference in your weight loss progress.*

**As we all have different sleeping times and wake times, the timing will differ from person to person. For example**

***Breakfast****: Your first meal of the day needs to be, and should always be, consumed within an hour from the time you wake up in the morning. So, if you wake up at 6 am you should have finished eating your breakfast no later than 7 am. This is because you have been sleeping for x amount of hours the night before and your body has been in starvation mode. Breakfast is indeed and always will be the most important meal of the day. The later in the morning you have breakfast, the more your brain will be under* *the impression that it may not get another meal for a long period, so it will store any food that it consumes. Have a full breakfast, as we are more physical during the mornings and afternoons, and we tend to be less physical in the evening and night. This way your brain will realise it has consumed more than enough food to exchange for energy and will not retain calories.*

**Lunch***: As you have had a hearty breakfast, you may not feel that hungry at lunch time. For weight loss purposes, split your lunch into two. Ideally, eat your lunch 4 hours after breakfast. The first half of your lunch should be consumed at 11 am, and the second half of your lunch should be eaten at 2 pm, (based on wake time of 6 am).*

**Snack***: Between 3 pm and 5 pm, if hunger strikes have a light and healthy snack, taken from the list of healthy snacks mentioned previously and below.*

**Dinner***: Should be eaten by 7 pm at the latest.*

*For modification, you could also split your dinner into two, but remember the latest time to consume food would be 7 pm. In the late evening, most of us tend to slow down and be more sedentary with fewer activities and less movement. This is true for our metabolism too, which also slows down.*

**Remember this is not a diet plan! It's a lifestyle change to your eating habits. You can see and adjust to your lifestyle and weight loss needs, as timing is everything.**

## PORTION SIZE

Is it too big or too small?

*Are you consuming far too few calories or is your portion size through the roof? Either one could be the reason for your weight gain. Portion size, like so many other factors, depends on the individual and varies from person to person. We all struggle with knowing the correct portion size to eat and the correct ratio of protein to carbs, fats and vegetables.*

**Here are two methods for portion sizing**

**Your plate**: *You can use your plate as a portion guide, but make sure this is a medium-size plate. The following measurement is for foods that have already been cooked and prepared. Note, this is only a guideline, as this could differ based on your lifestyle, for example, your exercise regime.*

**Protein**: *One-quarter of your plate should consist of proteins like poultry, fish, lean meat, pulses, tofu, eggs or beans.*

**Carbohydrates**: *One-quarter of your plate should consist of carbohydrates like rice, pasta, whole grains, or vegetables that are high in carbohydrates.*

**Healthy fats**: *Measurable by using a tablespoon, such as oil or butter.*

**Salad or vegetables**: *One-half of your plate should be made up of other vegetables or salad. Think* *of the colours of a rainbow, the more varied coloured salad and vegetables you have on your plate the better the nutrition you will consume.*

**Your hand**: *You can use your hand as a portion guide for foods that have already been cooked and prepared. Note this is only a guideline, as this could differ based on your lifestyle, for example, your exercise regime.*

**Protein** - *Use your palm size as a guide for your protein, have one palm-size portion.*

**Carbohydrates** - *Use your cupped hand as a guide for your carbohydrate, have one cupped-hand-size portion.*

**Healthy fats** - *Use your thumb as a guide for your healthy fats, have one thumb-length portion.*

**Salad or vegetables**: *Use your fist as a guide for your salad or vegetable, have one and a half fist-size portion.*

*When you are at a restaurant, order your favourite meals but consume half of the amount.*

## COMMON MISTAKES THAT CAUSE WEIGHT GAIN

### 1) Rewards

*A common everyday mistake a lot of people make is to reward themselves with their favourite cake or chocolate bar or a burger with fries after completing their workout for the day. People often tend to overestimate how many calories they have actually burnt during their workout. But if you think about it, that is the worst thing you can do to de-rail your weight loss goals, as you are only going to pile back on the calories you just burnt off and more. Try finding a protein shake that is low in carbohydrates and sugar but has an amazing taste that tantalises your taste buds, that you can consume straight after your workout. You can also try to limit yourself to a reward day once a week, where you can more or less eat what you want when you want, but only for that day.*

### 2) Only eat

*Do you consider yourself to be a mindful eater? Over 65% of the world's population are not mindful eaters. Mindful eating is when you actively pay attention to what you are actually consuming. The smell of your food, the texture and, most importantly, the taste. Instead, we are often busy watching television or on our phones or in front of our laptops working. Eating should be an enjoyable experience. Paying attention to what you consume will not only satisfy you, but you will realise sooner rather than later when you have had enough to eat. People that do not practice mindful eating consume about 25% more calories than those individuals that are actually paying attention to their food, and only their food, without any other distractions.*

### 3) Too many takeaways and at the wrong time

*It's time to be real and honest now! Honestly think about how many fast food meals, takeaways, ordering in or deliveries do you consume in a week? Whether it is within your home or externally outside your home, count it all. It's time to reduce that amount to once a week on your treat day. To make it even better, consume your takeaway during lunchtime rather than dinner time. This will reduce the effect of the unhealthy fats and excessive calories, and whatever it is they add to it that makes it taste so good! Eating your takeaway in the afternoon is better than in the evening or night because most people are more physical during the afternoon and less physical during the evening and night, therefore, burning more calories in the afternoon.*

## ALCOHOL AND WEIGHT GAIN

*This section about alcohol is not about trying to convince you to completely cut out alcohol in your life, but just to give you a better understanding so you can make better choices when it comes to alcohol and the different types on the market.*

*It has been reported that people throughout the world are drinking a lot more alcohol now in comparison to just five years ago. The problem with alcohol in relation to weight gain is that it is high in kilojoules (kJ), (kcal) also known as calories. If you look on the labels you will see that every gram of alcohol has 29 kilojoules or 7 calories, resulting in us consuming a lot more calories than we even realise. In addition to the additional calories, alcoholic beverages stop your body from burning fat to its highest potential. The other issue with consuming too much alcohol is that it does not contain any health benefits. As previously mentioned, it can affect your mood and your sleep over time, leaving you feeling more run down and stressed out. Furthermore, excessive amount of alcohol consumption can cause long-term damage to our health, increase our blood pressure or even cause alcohol poisoning. From drinking alcohol you can also develop heart or lung disease and certain types of cancer.*

*Like everything else, not all alcoholic beverages are the same. As we are mainly focusing on weight loss, here is a list of alcoholic drinks that won't pile on the calories when consumed in moderation.*

***The following is an estimated measurement of lower-calorie alcohol, give or take a few calories, depending on the brand:***

- *Brut (dry) Champagne 1.5fl oz comes in at 93kJ (calories)*
- *Gin, vodka, whiskey and tequila 1.5fl oz comes in at 97kJ (calories)*
- *Red wine 1.5fl oz comes in at 121kJ (calories)*

- *White wine 1.5fl oz comes in at 125kJ (calories)*
- *A small bottle of beer 12fl oz comes in at 130kJ (calories)*
- *Liqueurs 1.5fl oz comes in at 165kj (calories)*

*Avoid high-sugar mixed alcohol drinks like cocktails, as they are filled with extra sugar, syrups, fizzy drinks and juices.*

*Of course, you can still lose weight if you consume alcohol, just as long as you plan in advance what alcohol you are going to be consuming. Drink in moderation, ideally not every day. Choose a low-calorie alcohol beverage and stick to your planned amount. Remember, alcoholic beverages come with a set number of calories by themselves, so adding juices, fizzy drinks and syrup will only increase your calorie intake. This is the biggest mistake people tend to make. If possible, drink your alcohol straight, on the rocks, or add a slice of lemon or lime. If you must mix your alcohol, the best choice will be soda water, to keep it simple. To enjoy your straight or on-the-rocks alcoholic drink, you can add fresh fruit to your ice cube so when it dissolves it will give you that additional flavour with fewer calories.*

## ICE CUBE MIXES

Tips, try the following:

- *You could squeeze different types of citrus fruit in your water to make ice cubes.*

- *You could add one type or different types of berries in your water to become ice cubes.*
- *You could simply add a few stems of fresh mint leaves in your water to become ice cubes.*
- *You could formulate your ice cubes with just using soda water or just tonic water.*

*The choices are endless and, most importantly, yours. Using these tips, you could reduce the added calories and sugar to your favourite alcoholic beverage.*

*Remember that alcohol is dehydrating, so drink water in between alcoholic drinks. It's also always advisable to eat a meal before you start consuming alcohol. Have your last alcoholic drink no later than three hours before you go to bed.*

**Happy smart drinking***!*

## THE SWEET STUFF

*Sugar, sugar, sugar. It's in everything, it seems to be everywhere, and it piles and piles on the calories! As much as we actively try to avoid adding sugar into our food and drinks, there is hidden sugar in almost everything. Alarmingly, it has been reported that there are over 55 different words for sugar, which makes it easier for manufacturers to load up their products with sugar content and hide it away from the consumer. Some of the popular, and not so popular, names for sugar are dextrose, sucrose fructose, glucose, lactose, galactose, crystalline fructose, dextrin, ethyl maltol, maltodextrin, sucanat, barley malt, blackstrap and HFCS (high fructose corn syrup), just to name a few.*

*To confuse matters even more, sugar also comes in different forms, such as liquid, syrup, monosaccharides, and disaccharides (basic simple sugars).*

**Advice**: *Please note, if you notice any of those names and the generic sugar names on a food label, that doesn't necessarily mean that the item is a no-go, it just simply means you would need to pay attention to the sugar content for the product. As a rule, however, the lower the sugar content per serving, the better.*

*Also, on the subject of product labelling, if the sugar content is listed towards the top of the ingredients list, that's an indication that the product in question is high in excess sugar. A standard product label lists its ingredients from high to low, so whatever ingredients have the most quantity will be listed at the top and whatever ingredients have the least quantity will be listed at the bottom.*

**Tip**: *Try not to eat more than 23g of added sugar per day. Remember, less is more - less sugar, more chance to not put on weight!*

## SWEETENER OR NOT TO SWEETENER?

*Are you now thinking you're better off sticking with or trying out artificial sweeteners? I'm here to tell you that it is not. Researchers have discovered that artificial sweeteners are a gateway to actual sugar and can promote excessive weight gain. But it's worth remembering they are artificial, so they are made with very different combinations of chemicals. Some artificial sweeteners are better than others, but why risk it? There have been dozens of reports stating that artificial sweeteners are extremely bad for your health in a number of different ways.*

*It has been claimed that people who consume artificial sweeteners over an extended period can suffer from gut issues, headaches, depression and increased appetite, leading to weight gain, and could even increase the risk of cancer. Artificial sweeteners are widely used in processed foods and soft drinks, like sodas, powdered drink mixes, sweets and candy, canned foods, cakes and puddings, dairy products and jams.*

*Avoid the fake sugar in no-added-sugar foods and drinks because if sugar is not included, I can guarantee you that artificial sweeteners will be.*

> **Tip**: *Try pure honey, maple syrup or molasses as they have a lot of beneficial health factors and can satisfy your sweet tooth.*

## THE TRUTH ABOUT DIET FOODS AND DRINKS

*When your overall motive is to lose weight, you might automatically think to yourself that consuming foods and beverages labelled "no fat," "low fat," "sugar-free" or "low salt" would be a better option for us. But, in fact, that cannot be further from the truth.*

*When we think about it, if the ingredients that make the food taste great have been reduced or removed, then food manufacturers have to add other types of ingredients (i.e. chemicals) to make that food pleasurable. Processed low-fat foods generally have higher levels of sugar and other ingredients in them to compensate for the reduced amount of fat. Sugar-free or reduced-sugar products will usually have all types of chemicals added to make the product tasty. Diet foods are highly processed in general. It's vital to remember that you need healthy fats in your diet, as they help your body to absorb the fat-soluble vitamins A, D, E, and K and antioxidants from your salads and vegetables.*

*Not only can diet food make you gain weight because of all the added sugar, but it also removes any of the benefits from food that would normally have natural health benefits. For premium health and weight loss, avoid diet foods and drinks. Eat unprocessed, whole foods that are naturally low in sugar.*

# HOW TO READ YOUR FOOD LABELS CORRECTLY

*Completely ignore the health claims listed on the front of a product, as some can be misleading and downright untrue. Instead, pay attention to the food labels and ingredients listing at the back of the product.*

*Don't look only for the amount of fat and calories in the item. You should also pay attention to the recommended portion size per serving. The reality is that you are probably going to consume 2 to 3 times the amount of the recommended portion serving, if it's on the low side. Remember, manufacturers list their product ingredients by quantity, from the highest to lowest amount. So, you should pay attention to the first 3 ingredients, as they matter the most. If the first item listed is hydrogenated oils or any type of sugar, then you can be sure that it is unhealthy for you.*

***Advice****: If the ingredients listing has more than three ingredients listed, that is a good indication to let you know that that product is highly processed.*

## *If a product has listed one of the following in the top 3 ingredients, you should avoid it*

1. *High fructose corn syrup (HFCS)*
2. *Monosodium glutamate (MSG)*
3. *Hydrogenated oils*
4. *Artificial sweeteners like aspartame, sucralose and saccharin*
5. *Sodium nitrites*
6. *Sodium benzoate*
7. *Potassium benzoate*
8. *Artificial flavours and colourings*

*The best tactic to avoid unhealthy foods is to purchase whole foods and not processed foods.*

## EAT MORE HEALTHY FATS

*For years - and maybe your whole life - you've been told to stay away from foods that are high in fat. As a result, people consumed more refined carbohydrates, high sugary foods and beverages and processed food instead, resulting in a population of overweight or obese and unhealthy people. Now, however, we have become wiser and better informed.*

*It is universally accepted knowledge now that eating healthy fats - and even saturated fat - is good for you and has many health* benefits. High consumption of sugar is more detrimental to our health than fat.

## The best source of healthy fats can be obtained by eating the following foods

**Cheese**: Packed with fatty acids that have numerous health benefits. It's high in protein, calcium, and nutrients like selenium, vitamin B12, minerals and phosphorus, to name a few. All you need to do to gain all those health benefits is one medium slice of cheese per day.

**Avocado**: This is known as a "super fruit". They are high in healthy fats, a great source of fibre and potassium, and they have cardiovascular health benefits. Avocados can be eaten on their own or added to salad or even breakfast.

**Fatty fish**: Fresh fish, whenever possible, or otherwise tinned, like salmon, tuna, trout, mackerel, herring and sardines support and maintain a healthy heart, brain and skin. They can also help lower the risk of developing common diseases like depression, dementia and heart disease. This is because oily fish contains omega-3 fatty acids and unsaturated fats, with high-grade quality protein and other nutrients. It's advisable to consume two servings of fatty fish per week, with about 11 ounces per portion. People who consume fatty fish regularly tend to be a lot healthier than those who don't.

**Olives and extra virgin olive oil**: *Olives are commercially available in green or black form. They contain fibre and monounsaturated fat. Olives also contain oleuropein, which may help stop the development of diabetes in some people. Olives can be high in salt, so it's recommended to consume no more than about eight whole olives in one week. Extra virgin olive oil is the mother of all fatty fat, as it has tons of health benefits that relate to maintaining a healthy heart, lower blood pressure and cholesterol levels. It has antioxidants that can prevent your blood from developing oxidization, plus vitamin K and vitamin E. Extra virgin olive oil can be used regularly, but try to not use more than one tablespoon per meal.*

**Coconut, including coconut oil**: *Coconut consists of 90% fatty acid, which is the largest proportion of the richest saturated fat. People that consume high amounts of coconut or coconut oil are actually in extremely good health, as it has been reported that it can ramp up the fat burning process and actually improve your memory. Coconut fat or oil consists of medium-chain fatty acids, which makes them very different from other fats. When consumed they will go straight to the liver and help to improve your metabolic system. Coconut and coconut oil can be consumed every day, but stick to one tablespoon per day of coconut oil.*

**Tofu**: *This is a plant protein made from soya and contains polyunsaturated, monounsaturated, calcium, protein, amino acids, iron, manganese, phosphorus, magnesium, copper, zinc, and* *vitamin B1. It's suitable for anyone to consume daily, unless you are a woman with estrogen-sensitive breast tumours. If you are in that category, then you should limit your soy intake.*

**Whole eggs**: *We all know how healthy eggs are, but so many of us only consume the egg white when we're trying to lose weight. In fact, egg yolk has a lot more nutritional value than just egg whites. To get full health benefit, consume the whole egg, as they contain small amounts of almost all the nutrients your body needs. We have been misled to think that eating eggs will increase your cholesterol. On the contrary, it can help to lower the chances of developing cardiovascular disease. One whole egg has around 212 mg of cholesterol, which is 71% of the recommended daily intake. Eggs contain vitamin B, vitamin D, choline and lutein. It helps to maintain and support nerves, muscles, brain and liver functions. Eggs are a must-have for the weight-conscious, so consume them regularly, as they help to promote weight loss.*

**Nuts**: *Some studies have indicated that people who consume a small number of nuts regularly tend not to be overweight or obese. As far as health benefits go, however, all nuts are not created equally. It's best to eat a variety of nuts that are natural and only roasted with no added salt or ingredients, like walnuts, almonds, brazil nuts, cashews or peanuts. Nuts are packed with fibre, protein, good fats, vitamins, minerals and antioxidants. You should eat around 6-8 individual, but varied, nuts per day.*

**Dark chocolate**: *Dark chocolate is rich in cocoa powder, with the high level of flavonoids. Flavonoids polyphenolic, which* *are found in plants. You should select a dark chocolate bar that has a minimum of 70% of cocoa powder. You can eat dark chocolate in small amounts up to 5 days a week. Dark chocolate has more antioxidants than even blueberries! It's packed with nutritional benefits, helps to improve brain performance and lowers the chances of developing cardiovascular disease.*

***Chia seeds****: Chia seeds are small in size but packed with plant-based omega-3 fatty acids and both linoleic and alpha-linolenic acids. Chia seeds are also very high in fibre and very low in carbohydrates. They are packed with minerals and provide many health benefits. They promote a feeling of fullness, which helps to prevent overeating and aids weight loss. Ideally, consume 1 teaspoon of chia seeds three times a week. Chia seeds are somewhat tasteless but slightly sweet, especially if you're not consuming a lot of refined sugar. You can sprinkle them on smoothies, oatmeal, soups, salads, cakes and muffins, or you can make a thick, healthy pudding by soaking them overnight in almond milk or another plant-based milk of your choice.*

## PROTEIN

### *How much protein is enough protein?*

*As with just about everything, moderation is key. Protein does indeed promote weight loss, but it's crucial to understand how much protein you should consume in a day based on your personal lifestyle, activities and muscle mass. For example, you need to eat more protein if you do regular exercise and less protein if you don't do regular exercise. Your age also determines how much protein you should consume. If you are over 55 years old, you would need more protein than a 20-year-old that does not partake in regular exercise. Overeating protein regularly can store in your body as fat, which also could develop into weight gain, as well as lead to a higher risk of heart disease and colon cancer.*

*Do you know the amount of protein you should consume in a day? The daily recommended protein consumption by adult women is reported to be around 46g.*

### As a general guideline to figure out how much protein you should be consuming, do the following calculation

*Take 0.8g of protein per kg of your body weight. So, for example, a woman who weighs 140 pounds and does not work out regularly should have around 51g of protein per day. If you work out regularly between 3 to 5 times a week, you should consume around 55-60g of protein per day. Studies have shown when you eat the correct amount of protein for your personal situation, it can help you lose weight, especially around the stomach area. A known side-effect to your body and health if you do not consume enough protein in your diet could lead to edema. Edema causes your feet and legs to swell due to a build-up of fluids.*

## Signs associated with protein deficiency

- *Thinning hair*
- *Weak muscles*
- *Flaky and splitting skin*
- *Constant feeling of tiredness*
- *Bloating of the stomach*
- *Liver failure*

## Signs associated with consuming too much protein

- *Diarrhea*
- *Digestions issues*
- *Headache*
- *Dehydration*
- *Nausea*
- *Kidney stones*

## Foods that are a great source of protein

*Lean meats, poultry, fish, seafood, dairy products, eggs, corn, broccoli, brussels sprouts, watercress, oaks, hemp seeds, pumpkin seeds, beans, tempeh, quinoa, lentils, whey protein supplements, ezekiel bread and teff.*

## Meats with highest protein quantity: 1st Beef, 2nd chicken, 3rd salmon.

## List of high protein breakfast meals

1. *Toast with hard-boiled eggs*
2. *Toast with sliced banana and peanut butter spread*
3. *Oats (porridge)*
4. *Protein shake*
5. *Cottage cheese toast with avocado*
6. *Berries with Greek yoghurt*

*As always, consume everything in variation and moderation.*

**Advice**: *If you're at all worried or exhibiting any of the above symptoms, always check with your dietician, health professional, or doctor to get tailored advice on your protein intake.*

## TASTY HORMONES?

*When we think about it (and a lot of us may try not to), meat and poultry eaters are consuming hormones and synthetic chemicals, as meat and poultry are injected with hormones, and this has been happening for decades. So, when you eat meat, you are also consuming a percentage of those hormones, no matter how or for how long you prepare it. The majority of factories and farms all over the world that produce meat use hormones, so the animal can develop as quickly and as meaty as possible. The number of hormones that get into your bloodstream might be low, but they can be very detrimental to some people's health. This is because of hormone activity manifestation with the following carcinogenic effects, which causes a disruption to puberty and reproductive capacity. It also increases the chance of developing breast cancer in some women.*

**Tip***: Purchase meat or poultry that is not treated with hormones and, ideally, is also free from antibiotics.*

## PLANT-BASED & FLEXITARIAN EATING

*A plant-based world consists of not just fruits and vegetables, but also nuts, seeds, oils, whole-grain, plant-based dairy products, beans, and legumes. A plant-based world mostly consists of foods that are derived from plants with no animal source and no artificial ingredients. It helps to maintain healthy immune system, as plants have some key nutrition elements that you cannot get from other foods. The vitamins, minerals and phytochemicals in plants help to keep your cells healthy and your body balanced, so that your immune system can function at its best. Plants also give your body what it needs to help fight off infections.*

**Here is a list of scientific benefits for including plant-based foods in your world**

1. *Sustainable weight loss, as plant-based food is naturally low in saturated fat and free from cholesterol,*

*while being full of vitamins, minerals, fibre and antioxidants.*

2. *Lower risk of having high blood pressure, heart disease, and hypertension.*
3. *May help to prevent type 2 diabetes.*
4. *A longer lifespan.*
5. *Minimising the possibility of having a stroke.*

## *Flexitarian world*

*A flexitarian world combines a vegetarian plant-based world with the possibility to still eat healthy lean meats, fish and poultry, but just in lesser amounts and frequency. This can create the best of both worlds without limitation or exclusion, resulting in a win-win for your health and weight loss journey.*

## MICRONUTRIENTS

### *Are you getting enough micronutrients?*

*Micronutrients are very important elements that your body needs to perform everyday functions that maintain your overall health. They are grouped into categories, microminerals or trace minerals including commonly known ones (molybdenum, zinc, manganese, iron, copper, iodine and cobalt) and vitamins. The amount needed is generally small in quantity but can vary from person to person over their lifetime.*

## *The most important micronutrients are*

*Vitamin C, Vitamin B6, Magnesium, Zinc, and Vitamin E all play a role in supporting immune function.*

*To maximise your consumption of micronutrients, select the type of fruit you consume from different colours of the rainbow. To get a better understanding and what that actually means, I have listed the colours of fruits and their benefits to specific body areas and which can provide you with missing or low micronutrients.*

- *Orange coloured fruits: promote eye health.*
- *Red coloured fruits: keep your heart healthy.*
- *Yellow coloured: fruits prevent you from getting sick.*
- *Green coloured: fruits promote bone and teeth strength.*
- *Blue and purple coloured: fruits help to improve memory.*

*You can also get micronutrients from vegetables, which should be eaten raw (when possible) or lightly steamed to retain their maximum health benefits.*

*As another option, you could also take multivitamin supplements in liquid or capsule form to ensure you are getting all the micronutrients.*

## SUGGESTIONS, TIPS, AND ADVICE

### *Cook food with a steamer and or an air fryer.*

- *Using a steamer to steam your vegetables for 5-15 minutes (depending on the veg) rather than boiling your vegetables retains the vitamins and minerals that will give you the maximum nutrition. You can also cook fish and shellfish by using a steamer. You can even use a steamer to cook eggs (in their shell), meat, poultry and rice. A steamer can also be used to warm up some types of foods.*

- *Air fryers are fantastic for the weight-conscious and health-conscious, as you don't need to add oil to cook thoroughly and quickly, again retaining the food's health benefits. It's even cost-effective, as it cooks food quicker than a conventional oven. You can cook any of the following using an air fryer: French fries or chips, poultry, meat, frozen snacks or even baked goods. An air fryer can also be used to warm up some types of foods.*

## MORE GREAT OPTIONS TO CONSUME FOR WEIGHT LOSS

### *The best foods to eat for reducing bloated and gassy stomachs are :*

- *Asparagus, fennel seeds, papaya, ginger and banana.*

### *More great eats for weight loss:*

- **Spreads and condiments**: *Peanut butter (particularly the natural, no additional sugar version), mustard, ghee*
- **Herbs and spices**: *Arugula, chilli*
- **Snacks**: *Popcorn (plain), seaweed (plain)*
- **Liquids**: *Black coffee, apple cider vinegar*
- **Grains**: *Whole-grain oats, brown rice, kamut, chickpeas*
- **Dairy**: *Kefir, probiotic yoghurt*
- **Fruits**: *Bananas, blueberries, tomatoes, citrus fruits, pears*
- **Vegetables**: *Artichokes, peas, sauerkraut, pumpkin, sweet potatoes, cauliflower, cabbage, onions, bell pepper, garlic*

## TO THINK ABOUT/TO DO

*What lifestyle changes are you going to make after consuming all of the information you have received in this chapter? The answer will become clear when you finish your* **Analyse, Sort, Selection and Evaluate.**

*It's time to start making mini lifestyle changes, don't forget what we always say "Rome wasn't built in a day". Go slowly so your brain doesn't fight back to result in what it believes is the correct weight for you.*

**Congratulations, you have finished all 11 chapters of this book!**
**Now the real work begins.....**

# LEAVE A REVIEW, PLEASE

If you found this book useful and you enjoyed it, I would be extremely grateful if you could please leave a quick review on Amazon or on the website you used to purchase this book from:

## A HEALTHIER AND LONGER LIFE

AMAZING WEIGHT LOSS GUIDE MADE EASY WITH SUSTAINABLE MINI LIFESTYLE CHANGES FOR BEGINNERS. A MUST HAVE FOR EVERY WOMEN!

### H. A. SKYS

BIG, Thank you in advance!

## MY OTHER BOOKS YOU WILL LOVE - COMING SOON!

*At this point, I would like to make you aware of my 3 additional books (by H.A. SKYS) that will be available soon. They cover other further lifestyle changes that could help with your weight loss goals.*

---

# CONCLUSION

*I do hope this book has given you some useful information that will help you change your life, health, waistline, and overall weight that would last a lifetime.*

*To follow are the steps that you need to take to gain the body you always dreamed about.*

## *Analyse*

*You have now absorbed all of the information in this book and taken notes in each chapter as you worked your way through to give you an analysis of how the information relates to your own personal experience. It's time to start analysing your notes. It is recommended to read your notes at least twice to give you the best chance to really absorb the information you have recorded.*

## *Sort*

*After you have analysed your notes, start giving them a number rating. This means number each chapter or lifestyle change that you feel would help you to start seeing the weight start to fall off. For better understanding, here are some suggestions for guidance:*

*For example, a lifestyle change that you have already tried before but that didn't give you your desired weight loss result would be marked low (6/8). At any point when you were going through the book and retained a piece of information that you had a strong feeling might be an issue for you, should be marked high (1/8).*

## *Selection*

*Then, as a starting point, select one mini lifestyle change that you feel may be a key to your weight loss. It's important to only select one mini lifestyle change at a time rather than starting with 3 or 5, as you want to know which lifestyle change is actually helping you with your weight loss. One is the magic number, as it would be obvious to determine whether the change you selected is working or not.*

## *Evaluate*

*Remember you may see some immediate results depending on which changes you have implemented in your life. Some changes will show an immediate benefit between 2 to 3 days, whereas some changes may take longer within 1 to 2 weeks, or even more. We are all different. So remember that what works for one may not work for another. Our bodies' mechanisms differ from one person to another.*

*It's very important when you start to make changes to your life, you must keep notes on how your mini lifestyle changes are contributing to your weight loss goals. When you are moving from one lifestyle change that has not worked for you onto your next change, don't do it immediately. Give yourself 1 week from trying one mini lifestyle change before moving to a different lifestyle change. And of course, keep on doing the lifestyle change that is working for you.*

## *Final Thoughts*

*Whatever else you do, don't try to be perfect! When it comes to losing weight no one is perfect! Perfection is impossible and unnecessary just aim to do better today than yesterday. The best things in life that give you the greatest rewards always come from those moments that push and test you to your limits.*

**So, keep going, keep rising, keep believing in yourself! I believe in you.**

# RESOURCES

6 life events that can cause weight gain and how to prevent it. (n.d.). Today. Retrieved September 7, 2021, from https://www.today.com/health/6-life-events-can-cause-weight-gain-how-prevent-it-t199290

30 healthy smoothy recipes that can help your weight loss journey. (2021, March 2). Woman's Day. https://www.womansday.com/food-recipes/food-drinks/g1632/smoothies-for-weight-loss/

Annigan, J. A. (2018, December 9). What does food provide in the human body? SFGATE. https://healthyeating.sfgate.com/food-provide-human-body-6194.html

Bloomberg's global health index for 2020. (2020, June 18). World Health Net. https://worldhealth.net/news/bloombergs-global-health-index-2020/

Brennan, D. B. (202–04-08). What is too much water intake? WebMD. https://www.webmd.com/diet/what-is-too-much-water-intake#1

Brown, M. J. B. (2018, November 19). 9 tips to measure and control portion sizes. Healthline. https://www.healthline.com/nutrition/portion-control

Cohen, M. C. (2019, October 28). 8 best teas for losing weight and boosting your metabolism. Prevention. https://www.prevention.com/weight-loss/g29553192/weight-loss-tea/

Gunnars BSc, K. G. (2017, June 4). 10 High-Fat foods that are actually super healthy. Healthline. https://www.healthline.com/nutrition/10-super-healthy-high-fat-foods

Heger, E. H. (2021, May 28). 6 delicious, low-calorie alcoholic drinks. Insider. https://www.insider.com/lowest-calorie-alcohol

Holland, K. H. (2020, July 29). Are obesity and depression related? And 9 other FAQs. Healthline. https://www.healthline.com/health/depression/obesity-and-depression#if-you're-obese

How much water should you drink. (2020, March 25). Harvard Health Publishing. https://www.health.harvard.edu/staying-healthy/how-much-water-should-you-drink

Lawler, M. L. (2020, January 17). 9 scientific benefits of following a Plant-Based diet. Everyday Health. https://www.everydayhealth.com/diet-nutrition/scientific-benefits-following-plant-based-diet/

Lawier, M. L. (2020, October 26). 8 best and worst types of alcohol for weight loss. Everyday Health. https://www.everydayhealth.com/weight/best-and-worst-types-of-alcohol-for-weight-loss/

Nunez, K. N. (2018, December 7). Is it normal to gain weight during your period? Health Line. https://www.healthline.com/health/womens-health/weight-gain-during-period

Obesity and overweight. (2021, June 9). World Health Organization. https://www.who.int/news-room/fact-sheets/detail/obesity-and-overweight

Obesity rates by country 2021. (2021). World Population Review. https://worldpopulationreview.com/country-rankings/obesity-rates-by-country

Pietrangelo, A. P. (2019, October 22). The effects of depression in your body. Health Line. https://www.healthline.com/health/depression/effects-on-body

Pietrangelo, A. P. (2020, March 29). The effects of stress on your body. Healthline. https://www.healthline.com/health/stress/effects-on-body

Smoking & tobacco use- health effects. (2020, April 28). Centers for Disease Control and Prevention. https://www.cdc.gov/tobacco/basic_information/health_effects/index.htm

Stiehl, C. S. (2020, June 19). 30 hidden reasons why you can't lose weight. Eat This, Not That! https://www.eatthis.com/reasons-gained-weight/

Still, J. S. (2019, March 8). Thirsty? Here are 9 types of water you can drink. Health Line. https://www.healthline.com/health/food-nutrition/nine-types-of-drinking-water#TOC_TITLE_HDR_1

Stop smoking without putting on weight. (2019, January 18). NHS. https://www.nhs.uk/live-well/quit-smoking/stop-smoking-without-putting-on-weight/?tabname=smoking-facts

Stress. (2021, March 26). Mental Health Foundation. https://www.mentalhealth.org.uk/a-to-z/s/stress

Tobacco smoking. (2021). Wikipedia. https://en.m.
wikipedia.org/wiki/Tobacco_smoking

Veltkamp, K. V. (2019, May 11). Top 10 food ingredients to avoid. Spectrum Health. https://healthbeat.
spectrumhealth.org/top-10-food-ingredients-to-avoid/

Walsh, G. W. (2021, June 11). The best time to eat
breakfast, lunch and dinner if you want to lose weight.
Good to Know. https://www.goodto.com/wellbeing/
best-time-to-eat-breakfast-lunch-dinner-115224

What is the difference between stress and depression?
(2019, April 26). Alvarado Parkway Institute Behav-
ioral Health System. https://apibhs.com/2019/04/
26/what-is-the-difference-between-stress-and-
depression

When it comes to protein, how much is too much?
(2020, March 30). Harvard Health Publishing. https://
www.health.harvard.edu/nutrition/when-it-comes-to-
protein-how-much-is-too-much

Why people become overweight. (2019, June 24).
Harvard Health Publishing. https://www.health.
harvard.edu/staying-healthy/why-people-become-
overweight

World Obesity Federation. (2016, October). Healthy
weight loss. British Nutrition Foundation. https://

www.nutrition.org.uk/healthyliving/healthissues/
healthy-weight-loss.html?limitstart=0

Zumdahl, S. S. Z. (n.d.). Water. Britannica. Retrieved
September 7, 2021, from https://www.britannica.
com/science/water

Printed in Great Britain
by Amazon

11221610R00079